Your One Stop Solution to Get A Healthy, Slim And Toned Body!
Want To Slip Into Your Favorite Outfit?
Breakthrough weight loss ideas
Want To Slip Into Your Favorite Outfit?
Breakthrough weight loss ideas

Want to Slip into your favourite outfit?

Breakthrough Weight Loss Ideas

Table of Contents

<u>LEGAL NOTICE</u>

Chapter 1

Choose to Lose - Why Should You Lose Weight in The First Place?

"The chief excitement in a woman's life is spotting women who are fatter than she is"

-Helen Rowland

Okay, yes, this is an intelligent question. Why should you consider weight loss in the first place? Is being overweight an ISSUE? If you go by the consensus, obesity is an epidemic. There are many dissenting views on this as well but if you go by the generally held belief, yes, being overweight is an issue- a BIG issue more so because obesity is the mother of all problems. It may cause 1000 more problems! So, yes there is sense in losing weight.

A properly toned body adds confidence, makes your immune system strong, makes you stay energized, brings flexibility in body movements and above all makes you stay happy!

Now, some people find it difficult to identify if they are obese or not. There is an apparent difference between being overweight and obese and people must understand this difference. Many indicators can be used to assess the need for body weight loss. The most popularly used indicator is the Body Mass Index (BMI). Medical experts however are not unanimous on BMI as a standard obesity indicator since it does not take into account sex, age, race, muscularity etc.

The disputing views on BMI led to the development and subsequent popularity of other obesity indexes like the waist circumference method, body fat indication etc. The waist circumference method is especially effective since it takes into account abdominal fat. Abdominal fat deposition is more dangerous than any other form of fat deposition. Body fat index is also a better option over routine BMI.

Countless people around the world fall under the category of obese people and their number is only increasing. The sedentary lifestyle and crash diets have started to show in our health. The problem is all the scarier as childhood obesity is picking up. Let us take a look at some staggering statistics:

* On an approximate there are 300 million obese people worldwide.
* Obesity accounts for approximately 5% of the composite healthcare costs in some of the developed nations of the world.
* The population of obese children (less than 5 years of age) is approximated to be 22 million.
* Losing weight can have numerous benefits for your overall health and well-being. Here are a few reasons why you might consider losing weight:

* Improved physical health: Losing weight can reduce the risk of various health conditions such as heart disease, high blood pressure, type 2 diabetes, and certain types of cancer. It can also alleviate symptoms of existing conditions and improve overall mobility and flexibility.

* Increased energy levels: Shedding excess weight can boost your energy levels and make daily activities feel less tiring. With improved stamina, you may find it easier to engage in physical activities and enjoy a more active lifestyle.

* Enhanced mental well-being: Losing weight can have a positive impact on your mental health. It can boost self-confidence and self-esteem, improve body image, and reduce feelings of anxiety or depression associated with weight-related concerns.

* Better sleep quality: Weight loss can improve sleep patterns and quality.

* Losing weight can alleviate sleep apnea symptoms and reduce the risk of developing sleep-related disorders, resulting in more restful and rejuvenating sleep.

* Overall quality of life: Achieving a healthy weight can enhance your overall quality of life. It can improve your ability to participate in social activities, increase your self-confidence, and provide a sense of accomplishment and satisfaction.

* Remember, it's important to approach weight loss healthily and sustainably. Consulting with a healthcare professional or a registered dietitian can help you develop a personalized plan that suits your specific needs and goals.

It is high time we wake up to the intensity of these statistical facts!

Chapter 2

Exercising Your Way to Weight Loss Isn't It a Better Option Over Regular Weight-loss Pills?

A man's health can be judged by which he takes two at a time - pills or stairs!

-Joan Welsh

There can be two possible reasons as to why you are reading this page. One that you have already gulped down some weight loss pills and two that maybe you are considering taking on to them! If you have already popped some pills, well we cannot do anything about that but if you are still considering them for some reason, we would request you to read the following lines thoroughly.

The market is teaming up with weight loss supplements these days. The companies are promoting these weight loss pills as 'magic pills.

They may sound to be the fastest way to shed those extra pounds but actually, they may just screw it up all for you.

Not all diet pills are harmful. The genuine ones use natural herbs and botanical elixirs but others are intricate compositions. Phenylpropanolamine is a common drug used in diet pills. Studies suggest that this particular drug starts to show serious health complications after 1 month's usage or so. The basic mechanism of all diet pills is to suppress appetite.

This, in turn, causes a myriad of other problems like diarrhoea, nausea, irritation, sleeplessness, headache, heart attack, kidney failure, liver damage etc.

The side effects may range from being anything mild to severe depending on one person to another.

Furthermore, diet pills produce momentary effects. On discontinuation, the person usually regains the lost weight within a couple of weeks. What's the BIG idea?

Most people go by what a pharmacist tells them to do. How on earth can a local pharmacist over an experienced doctor? Neither should you go by what a pharmacist tells you, nor should you self-administer any drug. What on earth are doctors for?

We understand your desperation to lose weight quickly. But in this hurry may you not choose the wrong path. The 'Diet pills' path may seem tempting but you have to get over this temptation with as little botheration as possible.

Exercise your way to a better living guy! Exercising does not cost a penny. It poses no threats. It is a tried and tested means of weight loss.

It is easy and highly safe! Is there anybody who still thinks that popping down some weight loss pills is a better option than exercising? Absolutely! Exercising is generally considered a better option for weight loss compared to relying solely on regular weight-loss pills. Here's why:

Sustainable and long-term results: Regular exercise, combined with a balanced diet, promotes sustainable weight loss.

It helps you burn calories, build muscle, and increase your metabolism, leading to gradual and lasting changes in your body composition. Weight-loss pills, on the other hand, may provide temporary results and often require continued usage to maintain any weight loss achieved.

Overall health benefits: Exercise offers numerous health benefits beyond weight loss. It improves cardiovascular health, strengthens bones and muscles, boosts mood, reduces stress, and enhances overall well-being. Weight-loss pills, however, primarily focus on reducing weight and may not provide the same comprehensive health benefits.

Customizable and adaptable: Exercise allows for customization based on individual preferences, fitness levels, and specific goals. You can choose from a variety of activities such as walking, running, swimming, cycling, or strength training.

Additionally, you can modify your exercise routine as you progress, making it adaptable to your changing needs. Weight-loss pills, on the other hand, offer a one-size-fits-all approach and may not consider individual variations.

Safety and potential side effects: Exercise is generally safe for most individuals when done correctly and in moderation.

It carries minimal risk of adverse effects when compared to weight-loss pills, which can have potential side effects and interactions with other medications. It's always important to consult with a healthcare professional before starting any exercise or weight-loss pill regimen.

While exercise is a beneficial and effective approach to weight loss, it's important to note that a combination of healthy eating habits and regular physical activity is often the most successful strategy. It's always recommended to consult with a healthcare professional or a registered dietitian to develop a personalized plan that suits your specific needs and goals.

Chapter 3

How To Schedule Your Work Out?

"No matter who you are, no matter what you do, you absolutely, positively do have the power to change."

-Bill Phillips

First things first, you need to schedule your workout. The rewards of rational scheduling are priceless. Scheduling can be done orally but it is always better that you put it in ink. A written schedule brings about a little earnestness on the part of the follower.

Usually, people find it difficult to set a schedule all by themselves. If you are also jostling with the same problem, you may speak to a fitness trainer.

A trainer helps you to set realistic goals and kick-start with the fitness program.

Scheduling will take time but this time investment will pay you back in double. Planning is the first step of any activity. Methodological planning helps to achieve the desired goals more efficiently. As such, you must spare some time out and work out a fitness plan for yourself.

Fitness plans are highly personalized and as such your fitness program will differ from your friend's fitness program. You can't just pick up anybody else's fitness plan.

As an individual, you may have your problems. Your friend may be working to get rid of abdominal fat while you may want to shed thigh fat. You can't follow the same workout plan.

Is that right? So, you need to set an individualistic plan for yourself keeping in view your medical history, your goals, your abilities and your dynamism.

Depending on your goals, you will have to decide the exact form of workout for yourself. A good way is to devote different days to different body parts. This puts little strain on one particular organ of the body. Furthermore, it offers less scope for monotony. The otherwise repetitiveness puts off many people.

Many people have tried this integrated weight loss plan and benefitted from it. This is however not a standard plan. You may choose whatever you feel comfortable with.

You must also periodically evaluate your progress. Monitoring your fitness development will help you in setting future goals. If you think, you are somehow unable to reach the desired goals; you may consider some alterations in your weight loss plan.

The work does not stop with scheduling alone. You have to honour the scheduling as well. The scheduling should be such that it is difficult to easily reschedule, erase or cancel it.

Scheduling your workouts can help you stay consistent and make exercise a regular part of your routine. Here are some tips on how to schedule your workouts effectively:

Determine your availability: Assess your daily and weekly schedule to identify the best times for workouts. Consider factors such as work or school commitments, family responsibilities, and personal preferences.

Set realistic goals: Determine how many days per week you want to exercise and the duration of each session. Start with manageable goals and gradually increase intensity and frequency over time.

Prioritize consistency: Consistency is key when it comes to seeing results from your workouts. Aim for a consistent schedule that you can realistically maintain. It's better to have shorter, regular workouts than sporadic, longer sessions.

Find your optimal workout time: Some people prefer morning workouts to kickstart their day, while others find evenings more suitable. Experiment with different times to find what works best for you in terms of energy levels, motivation, and convenience.

Plan: Once you've determined your workout schedule, block off dedicated time slots in your calendar or planner. Treat these appointments as non-negotiable and prioritize them just like any other important commitment.

Be flexible: While having a set schedule is beneficial, it's important to be flexible and adaptable. Life can sometimes throw unexpected curveballs, so be prepared to adjust your workout schedule when necessary. Having backup options, such as home workouts or shorter routines, can help you stay on track during busy periods.

Incorporate a variety of workouts to keep things interesting and prevent boredom. This can include cardio, strength training, flexibility exercises, and rest days for recovery. Experiment with different activities and find what you enjoy to maintain motivation.

Track your progress: Keep a workout log or use a fitness app to track your progress and hold yourself accountable. Seeing your achievements and improvements can motivate you to stick to your schedule.

Remember, consistency and finding a routine that works for you are key. It's important to listen to your body, rest when needed, and consult with a healthcare professional or a certified fitness trainer if you have any specific health concerns or limitations.

Chapter 4

Exercising Does Not Have To Be All That Boring! - Interesting Ways of Exercising

Exercising can be fun and interesting! There are so many unique and enjoyable ways to stay active. Some examples include dance classes, outdoor activities like hiking or kayaking, team sports, or even trying out a new workout routine. Finding something you enjoy makes it easier to stick with an exercise regimen. If you'd like, I can help you brainstorm some specific ideas based on your preferences and interests.

"Exercise should be fun; otherwise, you won't be consistent".
-Laura Ramirez

There are a lot many people who want to exercise but they don't feel like exercising. Your workout has to be fun for you to be persistent with it!

Exercising doesn't have to be boring at all. It can be enjoyable. Here are some interesting ways you can make your workout routine more exciting:

Dance Fitness: Join a dance fitness class like Zumba or hip-hop aerobics. These classes incorporate dance moves into a cardio workout, making it both entertaining and energizing.

Outdoor Adventures: Instead of hitting the gym, take your workout outside. Try activities like hiking, kayaking, rock climbing, or even outdoor yoga. You'll get a full-body workout while enjoying the beauty of nature.

Group Sports: Participate in group sports such as basketball, soccer, or volleyball. These team activities not only provide physical exercise but also encourage social interaction and competition.

Martial Arts: Enroll in a martial arts class like karate, kickboxing, or taekwondo. These practices blend physical exercise with self-defence techniques, keeping you engaged and motivated.

Trampoline Parks: Visit a trampoline park and bounce your way to fitness. Jumping on trampolines not only improves cardiovascular health but also strengthens your core muscles.

Virtual Reality Fitness: Try out virtual reality fitness games that offer immersive workout experiences. These games make you forget you're exercising while you engage in virtual adventures and challenges.

Outdoor Circuit Training: Create your circuit training routine in a park or garden. Incorporate bodyweight exercises like push-ups, squats, burpees, and jump rope for a full-body workout in a refreshing outdoor environment.

Fitness Challenges: Set fitness challenges for yourself or compete with friends. It could be anything from a plank challenge to a step count challenge. These challenges add an element of fun and motivation to your exercise routine.

Remember, the key to making exercise interesting is to find activities that you genuinely enjoy. By incorporating variety and creativity, you can turn your workout into an enjoyable and fulfilling experience.

Aerobics, Frisbee, hopscotch, canoeing, skateboarding, skiing, horseback riding, hula hooping, dancing, juggling, and weightlifting- all require bodily movement and hence they fall under the category of 'exercise'.

The trick is not to make a workout look like a work!

Exercise means significant body movement. There is no need to necessarily hit a gym. The trend of aerobics is on an upward spiral. It is a great way to lose abdominal fat! Studies point out that a persistent aerobics session coupled with a proper diet plan leads to miraculous weight control. Aerobic trainers are easy to find and approach. They charge a very nominal fee.

It's great to hear that you're looking for interesting ways to exercise! There are so many options out there, from dancing and hiking to playing sports or trying out new fitness classes.

Finding activities that you genuinely enjoy can make exercise feel less like a chore and more like a fun part of your routine.

Is there a specific type of exercise you're interested in exploring further?

If you have a dog, what better? Dogs give their masters a chance to incorporate exercise/activity into their daily routine. Make it a point to take the dog out for a walk. You may begin with a walk around the house then a walk around the block and then further.

There are numerous interesting ways to exercise but nothing compares to 'Dancing'! A person does not have to worry about coordination or rhythm. Dancing is a great form of exercise and you will undoubtedly benefit from it even if you suck at it!

Gardening is another interesting activity that you may take up. It keeps you busy, gives you much-needed exercise and most importantly allows you to relish home-grown food! Then there are a couple of small things which you may choose to follow. Say for example you must always prefer stairs over a lift. You may replace your office chair with a stability ball! You may practice push-ups every day. There are many alike!

Okay here is an interesting fact! Bright colours like orange, red and yellow are known to boost appetite while blue particularly is a 'hunger suppresser'. People who are following a weight loss regime must see to it that they are as little surrounded by vibrant colours as possible.

Avoid being a lazy bum! Spark your creativity! Get more adventure; add liveliness to your fitness plan! A final word to those who say they don't have time for exercise-

Those who do not find time for exercise will have to find time for illness.

-Earl of Derby

Chapter 5

Emotional Eating - What on Earth is that?

Some people eat to feed a growling stomach while others eat to feed a feeling! If you fall under the latter category, you are an 'Emotional eater'. An emotional eater is a person whose appetite is not triggered not by genuine hunger but by a peculiar uncontrollable feeling or emotion (Hence the name emotional eating). On experiencing such a trigger, a person usually falls prey to junk foods. Let us study 'Emotional Eating' under certain specific heads:

* Emotional- Some people try to fill the void forcefully. They would eat to kill boredom, tension, anxiety, depression, loneliness, stress etc.

* Unwarranted thoughts- At times, people eat to counter negative self-worth remarks. They will find a pretext or two to eat. They will scold themselves for being thin or something like that.
* Social- Some people make an effort to eat more when they are around other people. The provoking feeling may be the apparent inadequacy to 'fit in'.
* Situational- Some people grab all situational opportunities. They would love to explore new restaurants and bakeries. Usually, the situational factors are associated with some form of activity.
* Physiological- These are somewhat logical of all. Physiological situations are triggered in response to physical hints. For example, a person would feel an increased appetite as a result of regular meals skipping.

If you suspect being an emotional eater, it is recommended that you maintain a diary to record what triggers emotional eating in you. Identification of the provoking elements alone will not suffice. You got to work on it. These peculiar emotions and situations turn into ghastly habits in no time. So, by the time you realize that you are an emotional eater; the problem has already turned into a habit. So basically, you will have to break the shackles of this habit.

Breaking free from emotional eating is not very difficult. The next time you sense being overpowered by a particular feeling, emotion or situation, control yourself till the time the feeling subsides. As an alternative, you may choose to engage yourself in any other behaviour.

It could be anything that captivates you. You may practice breathing exercises or you may take a bubble bath or you may talk to a friend. You will find the feeling gradually collapses!

Emotional eating refers to the habit of turning to food for comfort or as a coping mechanism for dealing with emotions. It involves eating in response to emotional triggers such as stress, sadness, boredom, loneliness, or even happiness. Instead of eating for physical hunger or nourishment, emotional eaters use food as a way to soothe or distract themselves from their emotions.

Common characteristics of emotional eating include:

Specific Cravings: Emotional eating often involves craving specific comfort foods that provide a temporary sense of pleasure and relief, such as ice cream, cookies, or chips.

Mindless Eating: Emotional eaters may consume food impulsively, without being fully aware of the quantity or even taste. They may eat quickly or engage in distracted eating.

Emotional eaters tend to find it challenging to distinguish between physical hunger and emotional hunger. They may turn to food automatically whenever they experience a strong emotion or feel overwhelmed.

Guilt and Shame: After indulging in emotional eating, individuals often feel guilt, shame, or regret for overeating or eating unhealthy foods, which can further perpetuate the cycle.

To manage emotional eating, it's important to develop healthier coping mechanisms:

Identify Triggers: Recognize the emotions, situations, or activities that tend to trigger your emotional eating patterns. This self-awareness can help you develop alternative strategies to deal with your emotions.

Seek Support: Reach out to trusted friends, family, or a therapist who can provide emotional support and guidance. Talking about your feelings and concerns can help alleviate the urge to turn to food.

Find Healthy Outlets: Engage in activities that distract or destress you positively, such as exercising, practicing mindfulness or meditation, journaling, or pursuing hobbies you enjoy.

Practice Mindful Eating: Slow down and pay attention to the experience of eating. Before eating, assess if you're genuinely hungry or if it's an emotional craving. Choose nutritious foods that can nourish your body and provide sustained energy.

Practice Self-Care: Prioritize self-care activities that nurture your physical, emotional, and mental well-being. This can include getting enough sleep, practicing relaxation techniques, engaging in positive affirmations, or engaging in activities you find fulfilling.

If emotional eating becomes a persistent challenge, consider seeking professional help from a therapist or counsellor who specializes in emotional eating and can provide specialized guidance and support.

Human bodies follow a natural rhythm of appetite. When a person chooses to override this natural hunger, he/she falls into the clutches of emotional eating.

Chapter 6
Coordinating meals and exercise

Exercising helps to solve only half of the problem. The other half depends on what you choose to throw in your body. There has to be synchronization between exercise and meals.

Coordinating meals and exercise is an important aspect of maintaining a healthy and balanced lifestyle. Here are some tips for effectively coordinating meals and exercise:

Schedule your workouts: Plan your exercise sessions ahead of time and incorporate them into your daily or weekly schedule. This way, you can ensure that you have dedicated time for physical activity without it conflicting with your meals.

Timing matters: Consider the timing of your meals and exercise. It is generally recommended to wait at least 1-2 hours after a meal before engaging in intense exercise. This allows for proper digestion and prevents discomfort during your workout. On the other hand, you may benefit from eating a small snack before a workout if you haven't eaten in a while or need an energy boost.

Pre- and post-workout nutrition: Fuel your body properly before and after exercise. Before a workout, consume a balanced meal or snack that includes carbohydrates for energy and protein for muscle repair. Afterwards, prioritize a post-workout meal or snack that replenishes your energy stores and supports muscle recovery.

Hydration is key: Stay hydrated throughout the day, including before, during, and after exercise. Proper hydration supports optimal performance and helps regulate body temperature. Consider having water or a sports drink on hand during your workouts to stay hydrated.

Listen to your body: Everyone has different preferences, needs, and tolerances when it comes to food and exercise timing. Pay attention to how your body responds to different meal-exercise combinations. Notice if certain foods make you feel energized or sluggish during workouts and make adjustments accordingly. Likewise, be mindful of how timing affects your appetite and make choices that suit your personal preferences and goals.

Balance is key: Aim for a balanced approach that includes a mixture of cardiovascular exercise, strength training, and flexibility exercises. Similarly, strive for a balanced diet that includes a variety of whole foods, such as fruits, vegetables, lean proteins, whole grains, and healthy fats.

Remember that what works for one person may not work for another, so it's important to find an approach that suits your individual needs, preferences, and goals. Consulting with a registered dietitian or certified personal trainer can provide personalized guidance on coordinating meals and exercise for optimal results.

Going by what you want to achieve, you may either chart out a diet plan for yourself or you may consult a dietician.

You may maintain your diet plan with ink or many online diaries help you to keep track of it. Online meal planners facilitate convenience.

Many people across the globe are sort of desperate to lose weight but can't somehow control the temptation of ingesting 'junk food'. Maybe these people are unaware of the innumerable 'Yummy low-fat recipes'. Tasty food does not have to be junk always.

Now, how to go about the diet plan? To begin with, a person must educate oneself on the calorie count of various basic eatables.

That will help you to decide what to eat and what to not. Every diet plan is developed as per individualistic needs but all diet control plans work on a single mechanism. They are required to take smaller but frequent meals.

They urge you to include more fruits, dry fruits, vegetables, cereals, low-fat dairy products and skinless poultry in your daily diet.

Let us now come up with how to coordinate meals and exercise. A person must not jump on to exercising immediately after eating. There should be a gap of half an hour to two hours between the intake of food and exercising.

The general conviction is that the larger the meal, the more a person should wait before exercising.

Else there are chances of nausea, vomiting and cramps. Health experts recommend that people should unfailingly take a carbohydrate-rich diet both before and after exercising. A high-carb diet is all the more necessary before exercising since it provides an immediate flush of energy.

A person must essentially abstain from alcohol intake immediately before, during and after the exercise program. Alcoholic drinks cause dehydration thereby leading to reduced coordination.

A proper diet plan and exercise regime are the only two ways to gain or lose weight. There are NO shortcuts to it and if you think there are any, well they won't work, we can bet on that!

Chapter 7

Warm-up exercises are indispensable- Why should you never skip a warm-up session?

A warm-up session is indeed indispensable! You need to prepare your body for the harder follow-up. As such it is important that you work up a light sweat before starting with any rigorous and strenuous activity. A person should not forego this vital part of exercising.

A warm-up session is crucial and should never be skipped before engaging in any form of physical activity. Here are several reasons why a warm-up is indispensable:

Injury prevention: A proper warm-up helps to prepare your body for exercise by increasing blood flow to your muscles and elevating your core temperature. This helps to loosen up your joints, increase flexibility, and improve the elasticity of your muscles, reducing the risk of injury during your workout.

Enhanced performance: A warm-up primes your body for exercise by increasing your heart rate and gradually elevating your breathing rate. This helps to improve the efficiency of your cardiovascular system, delivering oxygen and nutrients to your muscles more effectively. As a result, you can perform better with improved endurance, strength, speed, and agility.

Mental preparation: Warm-up exercises also help prepare you mentally for the upcoming workout. They provide an opportunity to focus your mind, concentrate on proper form and technique, and mentally prepare for the physical demands of the exercise session ahead. This mental preparation can enhance your overall performance and help you get into the right mindset for optimal results.

Muscular activation: A warm-up session activates and mobilizes the muscles you will be using during your workout. This activation improves the coordination and recruitment of the muscles, facilitating better movement patterns and muscle engagement.

It also helps to switch on the neural pathways between your brain and muscles, enabling quicker and more efficient muscular responses during exercise.

Gradual increase in intensity: A warm-up allows you to gradually increase the intensity of your exercise session. Starting with low-impact activities and gradually progressing towards higher-intensity exercises helps your body adapt and adjust to the demands of the workout. This minimizes the stress placed on your cardiovascular system and muscles, reducing the risk of sudden strain or shock to your body.

Overall, a warm-up is essential for preparing your body and mind for exercise, reducing the risk of injury, optimizing performance, and ensuring a safe and effective workout. It only takes a few minutes to perform a proper warm-up, but the benefits are well worth the time and effort. Skipping a warm-up can result in suboptimal performance, increased risk of injury, and potential setbacks in your fitness journey.

As you get down to start a workout, your muscles are stiff, cold and prone to injuries. A warm-up session prepares them for heavy doses. Light warm-up exercises raise your body temperature thereby lubricating the joints and tendons.

Missing out on a warm-up session would mean more chances of strains and injuries. Let us study the advantages of a warm-up exercise in detail:

* A warm-up session prevents injuries- Cold muscles are difficult to stretch. Warm-up exercises bring about flexibility in the body muscles. These exercises boost blood circulation. As a result, the chances of injuries are minimized.

* Helps to burn extra calories- If a warm-up plan is carried out methodologically, it considerably helps to burn extra calories.

* Helps to boost immunity- Yes, warm-up exercises do help to strengthen immunity. If you choose to forego a warm-up session, the body will not be able to digest the tough follow-ups. As a result, it will release huge quantities of stress hormones which may further weaken the immune system.

  If you don't want your body to be overflooded with 'stress hormones', you must never skip a warm-up class.
* Improved respiration- a warm-up session substantially stimulates respiratory rate. As a result, all - the blood flow, the heart rate, the oxygen supply- get improved.
* Activates sugars- A simple warm-up routine helps to activate body sugars.

A warm-up activity may take any form. Some people engage in low-impact aerobic activity. Others follow regular stretching. Yet others practice jogging/running.

You may engage in whichever activity you feel comfortable with.

Warming-up exercises are also known as 'loosening exercises. You must devote at least 10 minutes to a warm-up session before starting with any arduous activity.

The time length of a warm-up session may vary depending on the intensity of the follow-up session. Likewise, you must engage in 'cooling down' once you are through with the day's workout. Both 'warming up' and 'cooling down' help a great deal to relieve physical and mental stress.

Chapter 8

Slow And Steady Wins The Race - Be Patient, Give Your Fitness Plan Time to Work

How can a society that exists on instant mashed potatoes, packaged cake mixes, frozen dinners, and instant cameras teach patience to its children?

* *Paul Sweeney*

How true! The virtue of patience seems to fading away.

You did not gain this much weight in a flash of an eye and hence you can't lose it in a second.

Be realistic! Weight loss miracles can happen and they do happen but only if you allow them to work!

In the pursuit of fitness goals, it's important to adopt a mindset of patience and give your fitness plan sufficient time to work. Here are a few reasons why taking a slow and steady approach can lead to long-term success:

Sustainable progress: Rapid transformations may seem appealing, but they are often accompanied by extreme measures that are difficult to maintain. By taking a slow and steady approach, you give your body time to adapt to changes and develop sustainable habits.

This allows you to make gradual progress that can be maintained in the long run, leading to lasting results.

Avoiding burnout: Rapidly pushing yourself to achieve quick results can lead to burnout and a loss of motivation. It's important to prioritize rest and recovery, as well as avoid excessive strain on your body.

By allowing yourself time to adapt and recover, you can prevent burnout and maintain consistency in your fitness journey.

Building a solid foundation: Fitness is a lifelong journey, and building a strong foundation is essential.

Rushing through the initial stages of your fitness plan can lead to skipping important foundational aspects such as proper technique, flexibility, and mobility work. Taking time to focus on these fundamental elements will set you up for better progress in the future and reduce the risk of injury.

Gradual habit formation: Change takes time, and adopting new fitness habits is no exception. It can be overwhelming to completely overhaul your lifestyle overnight. By taking a slow and steady approach, you allow yourself the time to gradually incorporate healthy habits into your routine. This increases the likelihood of these habits becoming permanent and sustainable in the long term.

Mindset shift: Patience and persistence are key qualities for success in any endeavour, including fitness. Embracing the slow and steady approach helps cultivate a mindset focused on long-term progress rather than quick fixes.

It allows you to appreciate the journey and celebrate small victories along the way, leading to a more positive and sustainable mindset.

Remember, everyone's fitness journey is unique, and progress may vary from person to person. Rather than comparing yourself to others or fixating on immediate results, focus on your progress and trust in the process. By being patient and giving your fitness plan time to work, you set yourself up for long-term success and a healthier lifestyle.

Some people start with a fitness plan and leave it midway because they are unable to sense any significant progress. Yes, the problem may lie with your fitness plan as well but usually, it is the other way around. People give up because they don't find any apparent change.

Who can bombard this patience into you? Nobody but you! You have to tell yourself repeatedly that it is a workout plan and not a magical program. If there is nothing wrong with the workout plan, the results are bound to show up- sooner or later. The transition from an ultra-obese body to a perfectly toned body is a big one and it will take time.

In case you are not sure about the accuracy of your fitness plan, you may consult a diet consultant. You must consult an experienced weight loss expert before kick-starting your weight loss regime. The trainer will suggest you better ways to kill your desperation. At times, these feelings of desperation and impatience come from people around you.

You must identify such people and take steps to steer clear of them. Ignore if someone tries to pull your leg by saying that your fitness plan sucks or something of the sort. You are working your sweat off to get a toned body and you should be rather sure of the success.

Do not get fooled by advertisements and their unrealistic statements. The promises they make are a part of their marketing strategy. If you are not losing weight according to the assured rates, it's okay! You need not make much hoo-ha about it! Every person has a different way of action and reaction. It is normal, for heaven's sake! Do not worry about it!

The following lines encompass the essence of our living. Read these lines and glue-stick them in your head.

"All human wisdom is summed up in two words- wait and hope!"
  * Unknown

Chapter 9

Some Common Myths About Exercising and Weight Loss

There are several common myths surrounding exercising and weight loss. Let's debunk a few of them:

Myth: Exercise Alone is Sufficient for Weight Loss: While exercise is an essential component of weight loss, it's not the only factor. The diet also plays a significant role. You can't out-exercise a poor diet. Weight loss generally requires a combination of calorie control through diet and increased physical activity.

Myth: Cardio is the Best Exercise for Weight Loss: While cardiovascular exercises like running, cycling, or swimming are excellent for burning calories, resistance training (weightlifting, bodyweight exercises) is also crucial. Building muscle mass increases your resting metabolic rate, meaning you burn more calories even at rest.

Myth: Spot Reduction is Possible: Many people believe that you can target fat loss in specific areas of the body by exercising those areas. However, spot reduction is a myth. When you lose weight, you lose it from your entire body, not just one spot. You can tone specific muscles through exercise, but fat loss occurs uniformly.

Myth: More Exercise Equals More Weight Loss: While increasing your exercise intensity or duration can help you burn more calories, there's a limit to how much exercise alone can contribute to weight loss. Over-exercising can lead to burnout, injury, and increased appetite, which might counteract the calorie deficit created by exercise.

Myth: You Can Eat Whatever You Want if You Exercise Regularly: While exercise does allow for greater flexibility in your diet, it's essential to maintain a balance between calories consumed and calories burned. Overeating, even if you exercise regularly, can still lead to weight gain.

Myth: Weight Loss Should Happen Quickly: Sustainable weight loss is gradual and requires patience and consistency. Rapid weight loss can be unhealthy and unsustainable in the long term. Aim for a gradual loss of 1-2 pounds per week for sustainable results.

Myth: You Need to Exercise for Hours Each Day: While consistency is key, you don't need to spend hours in the gym every day to see results. Quality over quantity is essential. Focus on efficient workouts that incorporate both cardiovascular and strength training exercises.

Myth: You Can't Lose Weight if You Have a Slow Metabolism: While metabolism does vary between individuals, it's not the sole determinant of weight loss. Factors like diet, exercise, genetics, and lifestyle habits also play significant roles. Even those with slower metabolisms can lose weight with the right approach to diet and exercise.

By understanding and dispelling these myths, individuals can approach their weight loss journey with realistic expectations and adopt effective strategies for long-term success.

If you talk about common weight loss myths, there are countless myths floating around.

There is a host of wrong information reaching the general masses and a whooping majority of people labour under false beliefs and baseless myths. The following lines will guide you to distinguish between myths and facts.

When it comes to exercising and weight loss, several common myths can often mislead people. It's important to separate fact from fiction to ensure you make informed decisions about your fitness journey. Here are some common myths about exercising and weight loss:

Myth: Exercise alone will make you lose weight.

Fact: While exercise plays a crucial role in weight loss, it's not the sole factor. Maintaining a caloric deficit (expending more calories than you consume) is essential for weight loss. This requires a combination of proper nutrition and regular exercise.

Myth: Spot reduction is possible.

Fact: It's a popular belief that you can target fat loss from specific areas of your body through exercises that focus on those areas. However, spot reduction is a myth. Fat loss occurs throughout the body as a whole and is influenced by genetics and hormonal factors. Regular exercise and a well-rounded training plan can help decrease overall body fat.

Myth: More exercise is always better.

Fact: While exercise is beneficial for weight loss and overall health, more is not always better. Overtraining can lead to fatigue, injury, and a weakened immune system. It's important to find a balance that includes adequate rest and recovery to allow your body to repair and strengthen itself.

Myth: Cardio is the best exercise for weight loss.

Fact: Cardiovascular exercises like running, cycling, or swimming are commonly associated with weight loss. However, a mix of cardiovascular exercise and strength training is more effective for weight loss.

Strength training helps build lean muscle mass, which increases your metabolism and can aid in long-term weight management.

Myth: Exercise cancels out unhealthy eating habits.

Fact: While exercise can contribute to caloric expenditure, it's not a free pass to indulge in unhealthy eating habits. Nutrition plays a significant role in weight loss and overall health. It's crucial to adopt a balanced and nutritious diet alongside regular exercise to achieve weight loss goals.

Myth: You can't lose weight if you have a slow metabolism.

Fact: While metabolism varies from person to person, it doesn't eliminate the possibility of weight loss. While some individuals may have a slower metabolism, creating a caloric deficit through diet and exercise is still possible and can lead to weight loss. Adjusting your eating habits and incorporating regular physical activity can help boost your metabolism over time.

Remember, it's important to consult with healthcare professionals or certified fitness experts to get personalized advice tailored to your specific needs and goals. By debunking these common myths, you can make more informed decisions about your fitness journey and achieve sustainable weight loss results.

Let us begin with the most commonly-held myth about fats. Nearly 90% of the total population thinks that fats are bad. There is something called 'Good fats' and these 'good fats' are pretty good! It is 'bad fats' that you must abstain from. By no means can you say that all fats are bad for our bodies. Your body needs fat and you better don't limit your intake of 'Good fats'.

People who are following a weight loss regime also think that dieting is a good means towards desired weight loss. This again is a wrongly based conception. Come on, you do not need to starve yourself to death! Let us put this in bold so that it gets stamped in your brains. DO NOT SKIP MEALS! It is not about 'not eating'. It is about 'Eating right'.

There are some foods which you need to abstain from but there are others which are essentially needed by your bodies. Your dietary plan must be very flexible.

There is another set of people who believe that one may eat as much as one wants so long as what one is eating is healthy. Okay, do you agree that oatmeal is healthy? However, you add up calories every time you gulp down a cup of oatmeal. The thing is you need to limit your calorie intake.

The population of people who think that one needs to do a lot of cardio is also no less. If your protein intake is not adequate, your excessive cardio may worsen the situation. If that is the case, your metabolism will take a nose dive. This will shoot back.

This is the reason it is always stressed that you must carry out a cardiovascular activity under the supervision of an expert only.

To some people, it is a cause of worry if they don't after a heavy dose workout. It is very much possible to burn calories without sweating a drop!

Clear your mind of all groundless beliefs. Concentrate on what your health guide tells you. Wishing you a healthy life ahead!

Chapter 10

Weight Loss Regime Calls for Consistency - Being Steadfast!

"The second day of a diet is always easier than the first. By the second day, you're off it."

-Jackie   Gleason

The key is to stick to the chosen weight loss program no matter what. More often than not, people are at their full vigour on day 1 but gradually they lose that verve. The enthusiasm on day 5 should be as much as it was on day 1. For that to be done, you need to ensure that your weight loss program is interesting enough to make you stick to it.

Your plan must also be flexible so that it does not get monotonous.

Consistency is indeed key when it comes to any weight loss regimen. Here's why:

Consistency helps in forming healthy habits. When you consistently stick to a routine of healthy eating and regular exercise, it becomes ingrained in your daily life, making it easier to maintain in the long run.

Creating a Calorie Deficit: Weight loss occurs when you consume fewer calories than you burn. Consistently following a balanced diet and exercise plan helps maintain this calorie deficit over time, leading to gradual weight loss.

Stable Metabolism: Consistency in eating patterns and exercise habits can help regulate your metabolism.

Irregular eating or exercise patterns can disrupt metabolic function, making it harder to lose weight.

Preventing Binge Eating: Consistency in meal timing and portion control can help prevent binge eating episodes. When you eat regularly and in moderation, you're less likely to experience intense hunger that can lead to overeating.

Long-Term Success: Sustainable weight loss requires consistent effort over time. Crash diets or extreme exercise regimens may yield short-term results, but they're often difficult to maintain and can lead to rebound weight gain. Consistency fosters long-term success by promoting gradual, sustainable changes.

Psychological Benefits: Consistency provides a sense of accomplishment and progress, which can boost motivation and adherence to your weight loss goals. Seeing consistent results over time reinforces positive behaviours and helps maintain momentum.

Adaptation and Progression: Consistently sticking to a workout routine allows your body to adapt and improve over time. You can gradually increase the intensity or duration of your workouts as your fitness level improves, leading to continued progress in weight loss and overall fitness.

Stress Reduction: Consistency reduces stress associated with decision-making. When you have a set plan for diet and exercise, you don't have to constantly worry about what to eat or when to work

out, which can lower stress levels and support weight loss efforts.

Overall, being steadfast and consistent in your approach to weight loss creates a solid foundation for success and increases the likelihood of achieving your goals healthily and sustainably.

It is generally held that group weight loss sessions achieve easy and quick success. You may get together a bunch of people who want to lose weight and together you may work your way to weight loss. With the number of overweight people increasing, it will not be difficult for you to find a co-partner.

Furthermore, you must set only realistic goals for yourself- something that you think is achievable by you.

If you set too far-fetched a target, how will it be possible for you to stick to it? As such, you must set pragmatic goals in the first place. For that, you may use a BMI calculator. This will help you to accurately judge how much bodyweight you need to shed.

You must also keep iterating it to yourself – 'My weight loss plan is perfect and it will produce the desired results'. There is a thing with psychological belief. You got to just play with your brain. Every day when you wake up and every night before going to bed you must repeat the above-mentioned lines to yourself with full conviction. 25% of the work is done, if you care to believe!

Another major point of concern is to close your ears to what others say. Closing your ears does not mean refusing to listen, it means refusing to act. People around you will narrate their success stories to you in a very spicy manner. This should not however sway you over. You must use your sense of judgment. It depends from one person to another. Not all people show similar effects.

Finally, you have to somehow kill the temptation that forces you to be inconsistent with your weight loss program. We hope you succeed in doing that!

Conclusion

We are sure that by now you must be fully convinced of the benefits of a weight loss exercise program. The weight loss exercise plan works on a simple mechanism. The amount of daily calorie intake and the amount of daily used calories together determine your body weight. Every little thing that you ingest contains calories and every activity that you indulge in helps to burn calories. The more a person engages in physical activity, the more calories he burns! As simple as that! It follows pretty logically that a person can achieve a desired shape by indulging in any form of exercise.

Embracing a daily exercise regimen offers a dual benefit: not only does it aid in weight management and contribute to a slimmer physique, but it also serves as a powerful investment in your long-term health and longevity. The evidence is clear: regular physical activity has been linked to a multitude of health benefits, including reduced risk of chronic diseases, improved cardiovascular health, enhanced mental well-being, and increased lifespan. By committing to a consistent exercise routine, you not only sculpt a healthier body but also cultivate a future filled with vitality and longevity. So, lace up those sneakers, hit the gym, or take a brisk walk—every step you take today adds to the abundance of tomorrows you'll enjoy.

Incorporating a daily dose of exercise into your routine not only aids in weight management but also contributes to overall health and longevity. Consistency in exercise promotes weight loss by burning calories, building muscle, and boosting metabolism. Additionally, regular physical activity has numerous health benefits, including reducing the risk of chronic diseases such as heart disease, diabetes, and certain cancers. Moreover, exercise enhances mental well-being, reduces stress, and improves sleep quality, all of which contribute to a healthier and happier life. By prioritizing daily exercise, you not only strive towards a slimmer physique but also invest in a longer and more fulfilling future.

I hope you have a life filled with good health, happiness, and prosperity for many years to come!

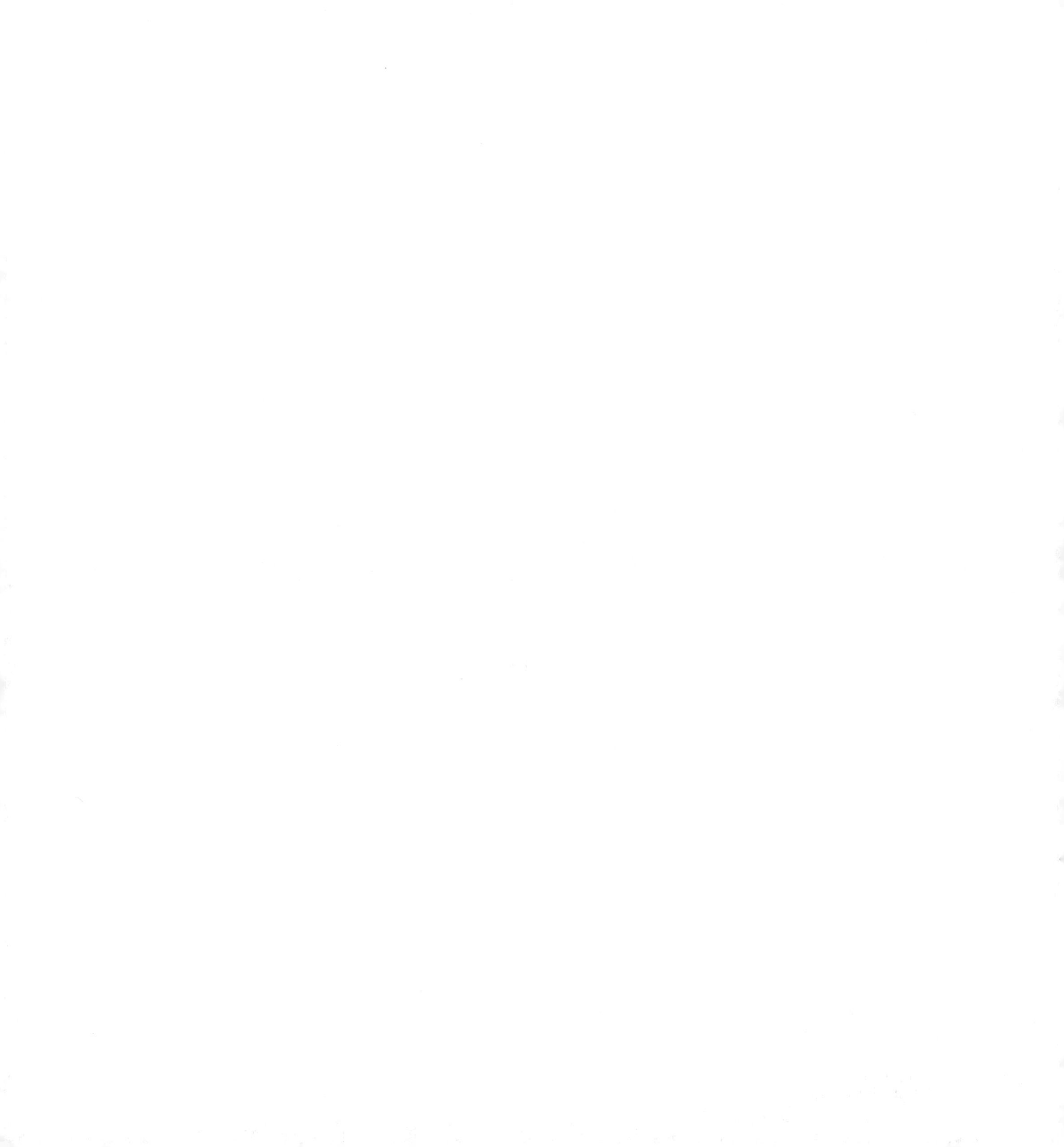